APPLE CIDER VINEGAR

The natural miracle cure for health & beauty in daily practice

TORBEN BELITZSCH

Torben Belitzsch

c/o AutorenServices.de

König-Konrad-Str. 22

36039 Fulda

Germany

CONTENTS

INTRODUCTION: FOREWORD

SECTION 1: THE EFFECT OF APPLE CIDER VINEGAR ON YOUR HEALTH

SECTION 2: LOSE WEIGHT WITH APPLE VINEGAR

SECTION 3: BODY CARE WITH APPLE CIDER VINEGAR

SECTION 4: FURTHER CLEVER USES OF APPLE CIDER VINEGAR IN DAILY LIFE

SECTION 5: MAKE YOUR OWN APPLE CIDER VINEGAR YOURSELF

SECTION 6: RECIPES WITH APPLE CIDER VINEGAR

INTRODUCTION: FOREWORD

The healing effect of apple cider vinegar has been appreciated for generations.

No matter whether you want to lose weight, have problems with your skin, want to do something good for your digestion, or as a natural alternative to conventional cleansers, apple cider vinegar is a multi-talent in many ways.

It is hard to imagine our times without vinegar. It is used to refine salads and sauces, to preserve vegetables, and it is vinegar that often makes meat tender and tasty. However, there are many other applications where vinegar makes life easier for us. In the household, vinegar can be used for dishwashing, as a cleaning agent and as a laundry detergent. In recent years, however, apple vinegar in particular has experienced a fulminant comeback.

Especially as a natural medicine, many people appreciate its excellent effect. It is said to help against aching limbs and headaches as well as digestive disorders. The reason for this is the high content of nutrients and the antioxidant effect. This makes apple cider vinegar the perfect treatment for a whole range of applications.

In the following I will show you what you can use apple cider vinegar for and what makes it so valuable.

APPLE CIDER VINEGAR - WHAT IS IT?

Apple cider vinegar is extracted from cider produced from freshly pressed apple juice by fermentation. The added yeasts transform the sugar of the apples into alcohol under exclusion of air. If the cider is now stored warm and open, the alcohols are converted into acetic acid by the bacteria. The apple vinegar is finished. A natural product which can be kept for a long time without any additives. The vinegar can sometimes be a little lighter, sometimes a little darker, and looks like apple juice from its colouring.

History

Apple cider vinegar is an old household remedy for the prevention and treatment of various ailments. Already the ancient Romans, the ancient Teutons and the ancient Egyptians discovered apple cider vinegar for themselves and used this miracle cure for many areas of application. For example, the ancient Egyptians used apple cider vinegar as a beauty product. They attributed the vinegar rather a beauty-promoting effect. They took care of themselves with it and bathed, were massaged with apple cider vinegar and even a kind of vinegar beer, called "Hequa", was very popular with the Egyptians. A few thousand years later, scholars have discovered that apple cider vinegar also has a healing effect. In the Middle Ages people protected themselves from the plague with apple cider vinegar. By drinking vinegar water to take advantage of the antibacterial effect of apple vinegar, attempts were made to counteract this disease. In addition, the healing of wounds was accelerated by dabbing affected parts of the body with apple vinegar water. Even Hildegard von Bingen, an important Benedictine and universal scholar, praised apple vinegar as a helpful remedy for intestinal cleansing. Christopher Columbus shall have carried barrels of apple vinegar with him on his voyages to protect his crew from scurvy, and Hippocrates, the founder of medical science and the most famous physician of antiquity, treated with it 2,400 years ago.

As you can see, apple cider vinegar has formative historical roots in medicine and medicine and is still a universal remedy for internal and external applications.

HISTORY

Apple cider vinegar is an old household remedy for the prevention and treatment of various ailments. Already the ancient Romans, the ancient Teutons and the ancient Egyptians discovered apple cider vinegar for themselves and used this miracle cure for many areas of application.

For example, the ancient Egyptians used apple cider vinegar as a beauty product. They attributed the vinegar rather a beauty-promoting effect. They took care of themselves with it and bathed, were massaged with apple cider vinegar and even a kind of vinegar beer, called "Hequa", was very popular with the Egyptians.

A few thousand years later, scholars have discovered that apple cider vinegar also has a healing effect. In the Middle Ages people protected themselves from the plague with apple cider vinegar. By drinking vinegar water to take advantage of the antibacterial effect of apple vinegar, attempts were made to counteract this disease. In addition, the healing of wounds was accelerated by dabbing affected parts of the body with apple vinegar water.

Even Hildegard von Bingen, an important Benedictine and universal scholar, praised apple vinegar as a helpful remedy for intestinal cleansing.

Christopher Columbus shall have carried barrels of apple vinegar with him on his voyages to protect his crew from scurvy, and Hippocrates, the founder of medical science and the most famous physician of antiquity, treated with it 2,400 years ago.

As you can see, apple cider vinegar has formative historical roots in medicine and medicine and is still a universal remedy for internal and external applications.

TYPES OF APPLE VINEGAR

There are a lot of different variations of apple vinegar to buy. The best way to buy apple cider vinegar is in an organic shop or health food store. Here you get higher quality varieties, which are obtained from whole apples and to which no chemical additives have been added.

In the traditional production mostly sour apple varieties from organic cultivation are used. In order to check whether the apple vinegar has a good quality level, it is best to check the bottle label. A note on the label that the processed apples come from organic cultivation and only whole apples were used, indicates a high-quality variety. Also the alcohol portion may amount to only maximally 0.2 per cent. A natural organic apple vinegar usually has an acid content of a maximum of 5 percent. Pay attention to the organic seal. This way you can be sure that the standards and conditions have been observed.

The production of apple vinegar begins with the juice of the apples, which is obtained by juicing. Then bacterial cultures and yeast are added to start the fermentation process. Then the sugar in the cider is converted into alcohol and later, in a second fermentation process, the vinegar is produced. This is done by so-called vinegar bacteria (Acetobacteraceae). The acid taste of the finished apple vinegar is caused by the vinegar and malic acid and gives the healthy "miracle vinegar" its unmistakable taste.

If, on the other hand, apple cider vinegar is produced industrially, only apple residues are processed and the acetic acid is artificially added. In addition, the artificial cider vinegar is pasteurized during production, while the organic cider vinegar does not undergo any pasteurization. The turbidity is therefore considerably lower and can be kept for a much longer time. However, pasteurization has a decisive disadvantage. The vinegar is heated so strongly that the important and valuable ingredients are only present to a lesser extent than in organically produced apple vinegar.

Pay attention to these differences in any case. This is the only way to ensure that you use all the properties of apple vinegar for your health. Organic apple vinegar also contains the valuable vinegar mother. The effectiveness of the vinegar mother for your health is not to be underestimated just like the pure apple cider vinegar. The vinegar mother is often used as a household remedy against colds and joint pain. Vinegar mother contains all the important nutrients and enzymes that make apple vinegar so valuable. The vinegar mother is a soft, jelly-like mass of acetic acid bacteria. If these useful bacteria are present in high concentrations, they can become visible in apple vinegar as dark streaks. The vinegar mother is harmless despite the strange appearance and can be enjoyed harmlessly.

In the end the following applies: with the most natural kind of apple vinegar you will get the best result. If you want to use the advantages of pure apple vinegar, you can also make your own apple vinegar. With the own production you have the guarantee that no preservatives, pesticides or chemicals are contained. How you can make apple vinegar by yourself is described in the book in section 5.

SECTION 1: THE EFFECT OF APPLE CIDER VINEGAR ON YOUR HEALTH

USAGE FOR YOUR HEALTH

As you can see from the introduction, apple cider vinegar makes a valuable contribution to our health. It can be used for both internal and external applications. It provides a positive benefit in many areas, from the prevention of diseases to various therapy options and body care.

Apple cider vinegar supplies the body with important micronutrients, minerals, enzymes and various vitamins. It contains vitamins A, B1, B2, B6, vitamins C and E, beta-carotene, as well as the minerals and trace elements sodium, potassium, calcium, magnesium, phosphate, iron, fluorine, iodine and zinc, copper, selenium. It supports and stimulates the metabolism, strengthens the tissue and keeps it beautifully supple and is very detoxifying for the body. Especially on the stomach, but also the remaining digestive organs such as the pancreas, the liver, as the most important detoxification organ, apple cider vinegar has a healing effect. Apple cider vinegar is able to curb cravings and it even keeps your healthy blood sugar and cholesterol levels in balance. And that 100%

natural! In addition, it is a very economical method of health maintenance. A bottle bio apple vinegar costs only approx. 1.50 - 2.00 euro.

In order to do something good for yourself, I would like to recommend you to consume high doses of apple cider vinegar.

However, the following should be noted: Never drink apple vinegar pure, as the high acid concentration could irritate the stomach. If you have a sensitive stomach, you should take care not to drink it diluted on an empty stomach. You could also try using apple cider vinegar in capsule form on a sensitive stomach. If, despite treatment with apple cider vinegar, the health problems do not disappear after a few days or at least have improved, you should consult a doctor or alternative practitioner.

It has been scientifically proven that apple cider vinegar contains everything that makes our beloved apple so healthy.

It is not for nothing that the saying "One apple a day keeps the doctor away" has burned itself into our heads and is supposed to suggest to us that we stay fit and healthy if we eat even one apple a day.

Allegedly 30 different vitamins, minerals and trace elements are contained in an apple. Until the late 80s that may have been possible in fact. Meanwhile we have several studies that show us that the food no longer contains what actually belongs pure. The example of the apple alone shows that the vitamin C content has dropped by eighty percent from 1988 to the present day. Only vitamin C!

As you can see, one apple a day alone can no longer be sufficient.

Thank God there is a form of apple that still keeps what it promises today. And of course we are talking about apple vinegar. How is it possible that the apple cider vinegar contains more active substances than the original form of the apple? This can be explained by the fermentation. Other important substances that are not contained in fresh apples are added, such as tannin (a tannic acid in tea and red wine), bioflavonoids (a pesticide that protects against harmful environmental influences), enzymes and organic acids such as acetic or citric acid. In addition, many people who suffer from an intolerance to apples (keyword: fructose intolerance) tolerate apple vinegar better, which is due to the production and processing. There are many healthy natural products that have a positive effect on our organism.

Apple cider vinegar, however, is more effective than most other natural products due to its versatile and effective effect on health. Scientists all over the world are fascinated by the effect of apple vinegar. It is proven and known that apple cider vinegar has an effect, but what exactly constitutes the effect is still not explainable today. Therefore one often speaks of the "secret of apple cider vinegar".

What is the effect of apple vinegar in detail? The following points have been proven:

- It supplies our organism with many vital minerals, trace elements, vitamins and minerals

- It makes the blood more fluid - an important building block for our blood

- Tightens the skin and keeps it soft and supple

- It improves the performance of the kidneys and liver

- Prevents the spread of putrefactive bacteria in the intestine

- It stimulates the metabolism

- It strengthens our immune system

- It promotes wound healing, as it has anti-inflammatory properties

- It slows down the aging process

- It has a purifying and detoxifying effect

- It refreshes, vitalizes and has a performance-enhancing effect and thus leads to more energy

- It regulates the cholesterol level

- Keeps the blood sugar level in check

- It relieves asthma

- Is balm for our nerves and helps with memory weakness

- It prevents calcifications

- Protects against osteoporosis

- Home remedy to support pregnancy

- Has a positive effect on the cardiovascular system

- Helps with diabetes

- It relieves muscle pain

It is remarkable that the active ingredients in apple vinegar can positively influence all these complaints.

I was able to see for myself that by taking apple vinegar water regularly in the morning, my performance and concentration could be increased a lot.

Overnight the body loses hydration and this deficit has to be compensated. Therefore, drinking is particularly important in the morning after getting up. In order to kill two birds with one stone, one creates the hydration balance with the water, together with the important minerals and vitamins from apple vinegar. This provides the body with the energy for a healthy start into the day, especially in the morning.

So add a large glass of apple vinegar water to your morning coffee. You can also add a teaspoon of honey to your diluted apple vinegar. The consumption of this remedy in the morning, on an empty stomach, supplies you with energy, enables an alkalisation (increase of the pH-value) of the body and gives you a protective shield against diseases. The numerous nutrients stimulate hundreds of processes in the body and help to balance the pH value. The pH value in the blood should be between 7.35 and 7.45. If this value rises or falls, apple vinegar can help to regulate the value. Apple cider vinegar thus ensures a balanced acid-base balance, important for the human body to function perfectly. According to many studies, too high an acid load has turned out to be one of the main causes for the development of chronic diseases and even cancer.

Let me go into some of the points listed above in more detail below to show you how helpful this remedy can be for you.

SUPPORT OF KIDNEYS AND LIVER

Apple cider vinegar contains an acid that is beneficial for the kidneys. Basically this seems contradictory, as the body should not be over-acidified. Nevertheless, apple cider vinegar promotes digestion and helps to detoxify and cleanse. The kidneys contribute a large part to the fact that the excretion of toxins, for example degradation products from the protein metabolism, from the body can function. In addition, the regulation of the water and electrolyte balance and the pH value in the blood is controlled by kidney function. These are just some of the many functions that make the kidneys an important part of regulating the body. Apple cider vinegar can help to positively influence this important regulatory function in the kidneys. As well as for the kidneys, apple cider vinegar helps to support liver function. Apple cider vinegar is one of the most helpful foods against fatty liver. It helps to remove the accumulated fat in the liver and supports the healthy function of the liver. Apple cider vinegar also helps to reduce inflammation in the liver and prevents the formation of stones and deposits in the liver.

Use the power of apple vinegar! The application is simple: Put 1 tablespoon of naturally cloudy organic apple vinegar in a glass of warm water and add some honey as desired. Best to drink one time daily in the morning before breakfast. Drink the apple vinegar water several months in a row to achieve the effect.

APPLE CIDER VINEGAR FOR A HEALTHY INTESTINE

Apple cider vinegar can also be used for intestinal problems such as flatulence and bloating. As already mentioned above, the efficacy of this product is based on its special ingredients. The condition is of course that it is a high-quality and pure product, so that the ingredients can unfold their full effect. Only in this way can apple cider vinegar have a healing and calming effect on the intestines and thus produce a balanced intestinal flora. It prevents the spread of so-called putrefactive bacteria and thus constipation and flatulence can be treated mildly, but consistently and permanently. The proven reason for the very good effectiveness of apple vinegar in intestinal problems is the high concentration of the ingredients in the vinegar. Much higher than in the original form of the apple. Compared to only one tablespoon of apple vinegar, it contains more active substances than if one would try to absorb the amount of active substances in the form of apples. Only essences are used for the vinegar, because this is the only way to ensure that the appropriate result is achieved. Many people (athletes, smokers, older people, etc.) need an increased amount of vitamins, minerals and trace elements.

Apple cider vinegar, if taken daily, helps to provide effective support for the supply of the body. It therefore acts like a gentle intestinal cleanser and thus prevents digestive problems such as constipation and flatulence.

In addition, apple vinegar is said to be effective against heartburn and reduce the feeling of fullness. Ideally simply dilute 1 tablespoon apple vinegar with lukewarm water and drink. About 15 minutes should pass between drinking apple cider vinegar and a meal. Who takes the apple cider vinegar however against heartburn should take it never directly after the meal. It is also important to always dilute the vinegar with water, because taking too much acid can have exactly the opposite effect and irritate the stomach and intestinal tract. It is also advisable to drink a glass of water afterwards so that the acid remaining in the mouth is washed away. Otherwise the acid would attack the important enamel of the teeth.

At the same time you should pay attention to a wholesome and healthy diet, because only in this way can one achieve the ideal supply for one's body in combination with the daily glass of apple vinegar water. Regular use can prevent flatulence and prevent constipation. Apple cider vinegar inhibits the multiplication of intestinal bacteria, which are responsible for the rot in digestion and thus cause flatulence and/or constipation. If you want to achieve the desired success, it is important that you pay attention to a regular intake; otherwise the gentle treatment in the intestines can have no effect.

CARDIOVASCULAR SYSTEM

The cardiovascular system supplies the cells of the organism with nutrients, hormones and oxygen. It also ensures that metabolic products are transported away. The cardiovascular system is thus one of the most important bodily functions. Even if the processes in the cardiovascular system remain largely unconscious, you can easily observe the effects. Cardiac tachycardia during anxiety, high heart rate during exercise, cold feet or flushing, all these are controlled by the cardiovascular system.

Apple cider vinegar supports the healthy functioning of this system. This is primarily due to its high content of potassium, fiber and antioxidants. The LDL cholesterol level (harmful cholesterol) drops when apple vinegar is taken evenly. Apple cider vinegar thus cleanses the blood vessels, makes the blood more fluid and protects the cardiovascular system, thus preventing strokes and even lowering high blood pressure. Apple cider vinegar, consumed regularly, causes a slight thinning of the blood, which is basically good for the health of the cardiovascular system.

RELIEF FROM ASTHMA

Asthma is a chronic disease that restricts the respiratory system. The disease can be caused by various causes and can cause severe breathing problems. So far there is no definitive cure for asthma. Only a relief can be achieved by various medications. Furthermore some remedies can contribute to the relief of the symptoms and as so often the best remedies are already found in the own kitchen. Also apple cider vinegar can contribute here by its useful enzymes to reach a relief for asthma patients. The enzymes help to reduce and break down the formation of mucus in the body. It is best to drink a glass of warm water daily with 1 to 2 spoons of apple vinegar to reduce the mucus and improve the inflammatory reaction. It can also be helpful to leave the apple vinegar water in your mouth for a short time before drinking it.

Another possible application would be to soak cotton pads with apple cider vinegar and press them against the inner wrists. All these applications, together with a healthy life-style, for example through an anti-inflammatory diet, help to improve asthma. For a while, do without industrially produced food and, as far as possible, sugar. A sustainable diet based on food that has not been processed causes the inflammations in the organism to be eliminated step by step by restoring a natural balance to the lipid walls of the cell membranes. Low processed foods usually contain little sugar, fats and salts. Therefore more vital and health-promoting substances are contained, such as vitamins, minerals, secondary plant substances and dietary fibers.

MUSCULAR PAINS

Many people suffer from muscle pain that can be more or less intense. The cause of this muscle pain is usually muscle strains or tears, which often heal by themselves. Unfortunately, this pain limits us in everyday life and especially during sports extremely and it often takes some time until you can fully use the muscle again. Muscle pain can often also be caused by chronic muscle tension. If the muscle has been permanently overstressed over a longer period of time or if a bad posture has become a habit, the muscle pain can become a chronic strain. In any case one should be treated early to avoid consequential damages. A further cause can also be that muscle pain can be a side effect for serious diseases of the musculature itself, the skeleton, the nervous system or other internal organs.

Let me briefly mention that I myself have suffered for a long time from muscle tension in the upper back and neck area as a result of constant stress in weight training. Through regular stretching exercises after the training session and massages I was able to get the pain under control. A valuable help to relieve the tension was also the treatment with apple vinegar for external application. I used the healing effect of the vinegar and took a bath with apple cider vinegar after the sport.

At first sight it may sound strange to use apple cider vinegar externally, but it was very effective especially for muscle aches. Apple cider vinegar can be found in almost all kitchens and is therefore quickly ready for use. Before you spend money on expensive prescription ointments or pills, you should definitely test the power of apple cider vinegar. In addition, studies have shown: Apple cider vinegar has an anti-inflammatory effect, in particular through the ingredient potassium, which calms and helps to relieve pain. The alkaline property helps to balance the pH value of the body and reduce muscle pain. Similar to lemon, apple cider vinegar, despite its slightly acidic taste, can help the body to settle into the healthy alkaline range and balance the harmful acids.

Fill a bathtub with lukewarm water, add 2 - 3 cups of apple vinegar and relax in a full bath for about 15 to 20 minutes. Repeat the bath if daily or every two days until the muscle pain disappears.

Even with bruises, haematomas or swellings, compresses with apple vinegar (undiluted) can help. The active ingredients contained limit the pain and help to reduce swelling. The application of a cider vinegar envelope is simple. Simply dip a cotton cloth into cider vinegar and wring it out. Then wrap the towel around the affected area and wrap a dry towel over it. Leave the envelope to work for approx. 10 - 15 minutes and repeat the procedure again if necessary after some time.

As you can see, apple cider vinegar has many applications - both externally and internally. An immediate relief of muscle pain can be achieved by a reactivating massage with apple cider vinegar. For this massage, pour warm water into a bowl, into a second bowl the vinegar (approx. 50ml) and moisten the affected body part with warm water using the cloth. Then apply the apple vinegar and 5g salt. Gently massage the salt over the painful area. You will feel that an immediate improvement of the pain occurs. It is exciting to see that this rapid reduction of pain can be reduced by the application of apple vinegar alone. A positive side effect of the external treatment is also that apple cider vinegar tightens the skin tissue and keeps it supple.

In section 3 I will go into the subject of skin in more detail and describe the advantages of using vinegar.

HELPS WITH DIABETES

Around 350 million people worldwide are thought to be affected by diabetes. A number that represents a dramatic increase over the last decades. Also in Germany there is a noticeable increase of the disease. Diabetes is therefore one of the most widespread health problems.

Diabetes is a chronic disease of the metabolic system, which is characterized by persistent elevated blood sugar levels. For those affected, this usually means taking insulin and the necessity of a strict change in diet.

Of course, it is clear that this will bring about a massive change in everyday life and that the side effects of insulin can also have a very negative impact on life.

So how can apple cider vinegar help as a natural home remedy?

. . .

Studies have shown that apple cider vinegar has a positive effect on the fight against diabetes and has proven to be helpful on several occasions.

Apple cider vinegar has a positive influence on the consequences of diabetes, such as the reduction of cholesterol levels and blood lipids. Immediately after eating, the income of apple cider vinegar influences the regulation of blood sugar levels and this is particularly helpful in the case of diabetes. The long-term and regular consumption of vinegar also improves the HbA1c value, the value that reflects the average blood sugar level in recent weeks.

It is important to ensure that apple cider vinegar is used correctly against diabetes. It can be said that the rule: a glass of water together with two tablespoons of apple cider vinegar has proved its worth. The vinegar is never pure, but always diluted with water to consume. Of course, you should be aware that a treatment with apple cider vinegar is only an addition to a medical therapy. If the blood sugar level is too high, it is advisable to take apple cider vinegar before going to bed, if you want to lower the blood sugar level for a short time, it helps to drink the apple cider vinegar water after eating. Occasionally, when taking this cure, the teeth may be attacked by the acid. Rinse your mouth with water and brush your teeth so that the acid cannot affect your teeth. Basically every kind of acid attacks the enamel. However, if you pay attention to dental care, you can easily avoid this problem. It is also possible that people with sensitive stomachs may experience stomach problems. Therefore, before taking this medicine, seek advice from your family doctor and obtain further tips if necessary.

All the health tips in this book cannot replace a visit to the doctor. If you have serious or unclear symptoms, be sure to consult your family doctor.

As described in detail you should pay attention to a high quality of apple vinegar to achieve the best possible results. This applies to the intake of vinegar to support the health of diabetes as well as to all other diseases mentioned.

In summary, the following points on the quality of apple vinegar are important and should be observed:

- Ideally, apple vinegar should be made from whole apples, not from leftovers or the core.

- The apples for the production of cider vinegar should come from organic apples and at best from regional cultivation.

- Your apple cider vinegar should not have been heated, so it is not pasteurized. Only a non-pasteurized apple cider vinegar provides the good enzymes.

- Your cider vinegar should be unfiltered, i.e. naturally cloudy.

- A quality characteristic is the presence of the vinegar mother.

- Your apple cider vinegar should not consist of juice concentrate and cheap vinegar.

- Apple vinegar may consist only of apples and not of other fruit or fruit mixtures.

SECTION 2: LOSE WEIGHT WITH APPLE VINEGAR

MOTIVATION

Many people fail to lose weight because they do not have the will or the persistence to succeed. The knowledge is available in principle, only the doing often prevents from the success to reach its goals. Keep up with the action and do not let yourself be discouraged by defeats.

 „In my career I have missed more than 9,000 throws. I lost almost 300 games. 26 times I was the one who could win the game and I missed. I have failed over and over again. And that's exactly why I'm successful." - Michael Jordan

In the following you will find basic tips to get your thinking on the road to success:

Tip 1: Find a goal that motivates you

To look at it closely, this seems to be the most important factor if you want to change your body sustainably. Having a goal that really excites you is the basic requirement to stay on the ball permanently. If this step is skipped, as most people do, you will most likely fail. It is crucial that the goal is your first priority, even before you lift a weight or start running.

Tip 2: Create rituals and change habits

Many habits are deeply rooted in the subconscious, so that you no longer perceive them consciously. While some habits help you achieve your goals, others hinder and slow you down. You need to uncover the obstructive scripts and replace them with new habits. This is the secret of how you can program yourself for success.

Tip 3: Take control of your thinking

Don't let bad, subconscious thoughts guide you. If you know your scripts that guide your thoughts, you can replace these counterproductive thoughts with thought patterns that are beneficial to you. You might know this, if something bad happens, you'll be thinking bad thoughts. This subconscious process is usually completely automatic. Try to get a positive attitude that will also positively influence your thoughts.

Tip 4: Find like-minded people

It is often very difficult to achieve a goal on your own. Create an environment with people who motivate you on your way to the goal. Which people do you spend most of your time with and are they the people who can support you in achieving your goal? If not, think about who can give them this motivation. Often, many have the goal of becoming sportier and healthier. Be it colleagues, family members or friends. You will do yourself a lot easier if you have someone at your side with the same attitude and motivation.

Tip 5: Find Mentors

Of course you can go the way through a personal consultant or fitness coach. However, a good mentor has its price, but is a good contact person and companion for detailed questions. Alternatively, there are the following suggestions on how you can find people to motivate you:

- by courses

- by books

- by podcasts

- by blogs

- in fitness clubs and member areas

- by a personal trainer

WHAT DOES APPLE CIDER VINEGAR DO TO LOSE WEIGHT?

In short, quite a lot! This somewhat lurid sentence, however, is absolutely true in the case of apple vinegar. The wonder vinegar, diluted with water, activates the stomach acid and also stimulates the metabolism. Thus the organism works more effectively and metabolises food faster. The result is a balance between stomach and intestines. If, on the other hand, the metabolism is slow, this results in faster weight gain.

There are, of course, many different opinions on apple vinegar and its success on our health and weight loss. However, it is certain that the fermented juice from apples is good for our general condition and our health. It provides us with a wide range of important vitamins, minerals, enzymes and secondary plant substances, promotes better blood circulation and prevents the growth of bacteria. Many factors speak for this slimming product:

- has a purifying and detoxifying effect

- stimulates digestion

- lowers the glycemic index and thus promotes faster weight loss detoxifies the body

- beneficial for fat burning

- causes a long feeling of satiety

- restrain the appetite

- stimulation of the metabolism

- Hunger attacks are prevented by stabilizing the blood sugar level

- serves the formation of gastric acid, which is necessary for digestion

- the contained kalium causes a dehydration of the body, which leads to weight loss

Nevertheless, even if you eat consciously and consume apple cider vinegar every day, make sure you get enough exercise and sports activity. Because only the combination of a healthy diet and enough exercise brings success for a healthy life.

APPLE CIDER VINEGAR DIET

Basically it must be pointed out that healthy weight loss is always advisable. Especially for health reasons, such as diabetes mentioned above, weight loss makes health sense.

The German Nutrition Society (Deutsche Gesellschaft für Ernährung) rightly confirms through studies: the calories consumed during the entire day and therefore also the total energy balance is decisive for body weight. If you supply more energy than you consume, you will not achieve success on the scales.

In the morning after getting up, drink a glass of water diluted with apple vinegar (approx. 1 tablespoon). Please do not think that the dream body can be achieved by taking cider vinegar in the morning alone. It should also be considered that the combination of apple cider vinegar, plus sport, plus a healthy diet (ideally high in protein) can achieve the goal. Please consider apple cider vinegar as a supporting measure in a number of other factors:

- Avoid foods with a high fat content as much as possible (if possible, use healthy, unsaturated fats such as fish oils, avocados, peanuts or peanut butter, rapeseed oil and olive oil for your fat requirements).

- Eat lots of vegetables and fruit, the main focus should be on vegetables. As a rule of general principle you should remember: about two thirds of vegetables and ideally one third of proteins with every meal.

- Season your food with as little salt as possible.

- Avoid alcohol.

- Sleep is important for our regeneration. Make sure you get enough sleep.

Do without the so-called "crash diet". It has been shown that a radical weight loss is firstly not healthy and secondly the yo-yo effect is very likely in the case of rapid weight loss. In order to achieve a long-term effect and to achieve and maintain your desired weight, you should refrain from these radical measures.

There are a number of healthy diets that bring the desired success and do not harm the body. The apple cider vinegar diet is definitely one of them!

A diet with apple vinegar is the most natural and cheapest way to lose weight. This diet is easy to manage and requires only a minimum of time and organizational effort. The above mentioned effects can be achieved by drinking a glass of apple vinegar diluted with water about a quarter of an hour before each meal. The apple vinegar drink is the basis of this diet.

The following is my recommended recipe for making the apple vinegar drink:

- Mix a glass of lukewarm water with two teaspoons of apple vinegar and add some honey or apple juice as desired.

Drink the apple vinegar drink before each meal and additionally before going to sleep to promote fat burning and digestion during sleep. It can also be drunk between meals to alleviate an upcoming feeling of hunger. In the cider vinegar diet you should consume a maximum of 1200 calories a day, depending on your daily energy consumption. Obtain the calories mainly from vegetables, fruit and whole grain cereals. Please note, as already described, that a balanced diet and enough exercise should always be an important part of life.

Basically there is no specified time how long you should follow the diet. It basically depends on how much weight you want to lose personally. Nevertheless, try to follow the diet for 4 - 5 weeks in order to achieve long-term weight loss. You will notice that the apple vinegar makes you feel fitter and more balanced, and you also lose weight. On average, the apple You can see that this diet is not a fast diet, but it is healthy and on the other hand you profit from a long-term success. The so-called yo-yo effect is eliminated and you consciously get used to a healthy and balanced diet.

It is all the easier to adapt to a new nutritional situation if you replace old habits with new, healthy rituals and let them become part of everyday life. Your subconscious automatically adapts to this new situation and your thinking and acting will have a positive influence after some time. Prefer this healthy variation of a diet to a crash diet because, in addition to weight loss, you will also change your attitude towards healthy living.

APPLE CIDER VINEGAR CURE - DETOX / DETOXIFICATION WITH APPLE CIDER VINEGAR

A apple cider vinegar cure is in contrast to a apple cider vinegar diet somewhat more differentiated to see. With this form one renounces completely, several days, on solid food, so that the body can purify and detoxify at the same time. After this time, the intake of solid food in the daily diet plan is slowly resumed. You could therefore consider the apple vinegar cure as a kind of detox diet or as therapeutic fasting.

The special effect of pectin has already been confirmed by medicine. It is a component of apple vinegar and helps to attract toxic substances in the body and to excrete them quickly. Another positive side effect of pectin is that it reduces cravings. It gives the body a feeling of fullness in a gentle way and thus helps to get through the cure more easily. Simply drink diluted apple cider vinegar throughout the day and you will get a feeling of hunger under control. In addition to pectin, sulphur is also contained. Sulphur also helps with detoxification and helps to stimulate the liver to process and eliminate toxins more quickly.

A further advantage of apple cider vinegar in comparison to

fruit juices is that it contains only a fraction of calories, but all the more important nutrients. A lack of these nutrients is thus prevented, while at the same time solid food is avoided. It is therefore perfect for losing weight.

If you decide to take the apple cider vinegar cure, you should do this in two phases; a fasting phase followed by a phase in which the body is slowly supplied with solid food again. During the fasting phase, you should refrain from eating solid food and consume a corresponding amount of diluted apple vinegar. The duration of this fasting period can be between a few days and 1-2 weeks. Just pay attention to how you tolerate the cure and how you feel about it. Drink the apple cider vinegar drink several times a day instead of meals and at will if a feeling of hunger arises. Furthermore it is necessary to drink enough liquid in the form of water, unsweetened tea and clear soups to avoid dehydration. Pay attention to your well-being as written above. However, if you experience stomach pain or discomfort, discontinue the cider vinegar treatment and talk to your doctor.

Advantages of the apple cider vinegar cure:

- the body is purified during the fasting phase

- Toxins are excreted

- significant weight loss, connective tissue and fat cells are relieved

- inner purification has a rejuvenating effect on the body cells

- defensive forces are strengthened

- Cellulite is alleviated or disappears completely, the skin becomes firmer

- more energy, well-being and health

- Deposits on digestive organs are liberated

After the fasting cure it is important to gradually get the body used to solid food again. Also make sure that you maintain a healthy diet. This should become a routine and lifestyle for you. For the first few days after fasting you should eat food that is easily digestible. For example: Crispbread, rusk, vegetables, fruit, soups and muesli. Gradually you can also eat foods that take a little longer to digest, such as whole grain bread, chicken meat and dairy products.

In the last phase of the cure, apple cider vinegar remains an important component of your diet. Sometimes it can happen quickly that the so-called yo-yo effect can occur as a result of cravings and you fall back into your old behaviour patterns.

To prevent this, apple cider vinegar serves as an aid to curb your appetite. So drink a glass of diluted apple cider vinegar half an hour before your meal. Stick to this tip to finish the cure successfully until the end. You can of course continue to drink the diluted apple cider vinegar at any time, independent of a fasting cure. This also helps you to keep your weight in the long run and to feel fit and healthier.

SECTION 3: BODY CARE WITH APPLE CIDER VINEGAR

HAIR CARE

Hair can quickly become matt and dull due to many external influences or excessive or incorrect care. The reason for this is the protective layer of the hair, which is damaged by an increased load. You can imagine the protective layer of the hair like small dandruff that lies on top of each other like roof tiles on the hair and thus protects the hair. If this protection is broken, the scales lose their structure and the hair looks weak and no longer healthy.

Apple vinegar acetic acid now causes the flakes to lie together smooth again and the hair to look healthy and shiny.

Mix apple vinegar with water to apply a conditioner after shampooing. Leave the conditioner in the hair after washing and do not wash it out. The active ingredients of apple vinegar have the possibility to get into the hair and scalp. Apple cider vinegar removes the remains of shampoo, soap and grease. The acid in cider vinegar additionally disinfects and fights bacteria and fungi, cleaning the pores in the hair structure. The big disadvantage of shampoos is that the pH level is changed. Malacetic acid balances out this pH level, making greasy hair pleasantly soft and shiny. The partly unpleasant smell will evaporate within a short time after drying. Just try this type of conditioner and you will see that the result will be velvety soft and shiny hair.

The use of this natural conditioner is very simple. One part cider vinegar is mixed with two parts water. After shampooing, the conditioner is poured over the hair and massaged into the hair tips and scalp. Then simply dry the hair as usual with a towel. The rinse as already described does not need to be washed out. Repeat the apple vinegar rinse after each hair wash or as often as you like. In contrast to conditioner from the drugstore, the apple cider vinegar conditioner is absolutely natural and therefore permanently applicable.

Basically the cure is suitable for most hair types. The conditioner can be used for both short and long hair and helps dry tips to become soft and supple again. However, if you have coloured hair, it makes sense to test a single strand of hair before rinsing, as the acid in apple vinegar can bleach the colour.

Advantages of an apple vinegar conditioner for hair care:

- Reduces dandruff and itching

- Dry hair becomes soft and shiny again

- Hair structure will be smoothed out

- Hair splitting is reduced by the application of apple vinegar

- Hair loss can be positively counteracted

- The pores of greasy hair will be cleaned and thus nicely cared for again

Finally, I can say that I am very enthusiastic about the apple cider vinegar conditioner. After a longer application my damaged hair structure has regenerated (due to too frequent hair washing) and the dandruff has been significantly reduced. In addition, my hair became shiny and handy and noticeably softer. In short, it has been shown that apple cider vinegar can help with a variety of hair problems and regain the original, powerful hair.

SKIN AND FACE CARE

In the following I would like to describe the effect of apple cider vinegar on the skin. To give you tips for the application with impure, oily as well as mature skin and to point out the advantages of this natural care.

The effect of apple vinegar on the skin is varied and effective. Why buy expensive cosmetic products that also contain chemical additives and are often tested on animals? Of course it takes time for the skin to adjust to cider vinegar care, but it is absolutely to your advantage. To say that the skin will thank you for it.

The fruit acid in apple vinegar reduces the fine pores of the skin and thus reduces sebum production. In addition, blood circulation will be stimulated, the skin tightened and skin aging counteracted. The application is therefore also very suitable for mature skin. The fresh apple scent vitalizes and refreshes the skin additionally. If you suffer from itchy and irritated skin, malacetic acid helps to alleviate inflammation and itching.

Apple cider vinegar for impure skin:

One of the most important factors with impure skin is in any case the thorough cleaning before you start with the care. In order to remove dead skin flakes, the application of an apple vinegar peeling is suitable in addition to conventional peeling. You will need a towel, a cotton cloth, warm water and 2 tablespoons of apple cider vinegar. First, soak the towel in warm water and place it on the cleansed face for a few minutes. The aim is for the pores to open through the warm water in order to be prepared for the peeling. Then mix approx. 0.5 litres of warm water with the vinegar and soak the cotton cloth in it. Place the towel on the face, moistened with vinegar water, and place the terry towel over it. After about 5 minutes the towels can be removed and the face washed with warm water.

Apple cider vinegar to treat oily skin:

If you clean your face regularly with apple cider vinegar, you will automatically prevent blackheads and pimples. The apple cider vinegar causes the fine pores to contract and thus prevents excessive sebum production. In addition, the acid kills the bacterias.

In the following you will find a recipe and the application for a facial tonic based on apple cider vinegar:

- Mix 50 ml mineral water with 50 ml apple vinegar in a bottle

- After cleansing the face, dab on the apple vinegar facial tonic with a cotton wool pad

- No washing off of the mixture is necessary, because the smell disappears after a few minutes

- Usage: 1-2 times daily

Apple cider vinegar for mature skin:

Even with mature, pale skin apple cider vinegar is very well applicable. You can rub organic apple cider vinegar on your body and face at any time after taking a shower. This natural application of a body lotion promotes the blood circulation of the skin and tightens it additionally. However, it is important to always dilute apple vinegar with water to prevent allergic reactions.

HAND CARE

To take care of your hands it is recommended to make your own natural hand cream. You need:

- 2 tablespoons organic apple cider vinegar

- 1 egg yolk

- 4 tablespoons olive oil

All the ingredients have to be mixed together: first the egg yolk has to be beaten until foamy and then the olive oil to be added. Finally, add the apple cider vinegar and mix the cream to a smooth mass. You can use the hand cream immediately. The hands will be soft after application and look wonderfully well cared after.

FOOT CARE/ATHLETE'S FOOT

The wonder drug cider vinegar is even able to alleviate complaints of the feet and partly even completely eliminate them. Besides, apple cider vinegar can also have a preventive effect and promote blood circulation. Application examples are:

Athlete's foot: If you suffer from athlete's foot, apple cider vinegar can help fight the athlete's foot. Soak your feet in an apple cider vinegar water foot bath and rub the feet with apple cider vinegar. To intensify the whole application you can soak socks in apple vinegar water and wring them out well. Put on dry socks and leave them on overnight so that the active ingredients can be absorbed well.

Dry feet: You can get dry and chapped feet soft and supple again with an apple vinegar treatment. Also here the application is very easy. Simply mix one part apple cider vinegar with two parts water and enjoy the foot bath. Be sure to apply it regularly, as this is the only way to achieve the desired result.

Perspiring feet: In order to achieve a regulation of the sweat production at the feet, one can maintain the feet, similarly as with the above-mentioned applications, by a regular foot bath. It also helps to rub the feet with undiluted vinegar. The acid in apple vinegar disinfects and prevents the formation of new bacteria. The smell will be eliminated.

Corneal removal: After a foot bath with approx. 35 degrees warm apple vinegar water, the cornea is soft and dead skin cells are removed. After the foot bath you can easily remove the cornea.

Tired/swollen feet: When you perform a physically demanding activity in a standing position, you often have tired and heavy feet. Apple cider vinegar alleviates these complaints and gives rest and recovery back to the feet. In the evening, treat yourself to a relaxing foot bath with one part cider vinegar and two parts warm water. If you wish, you can also add sea salt. This ensures that the feet are simultaneously subjected to a peeling and become beautifully supple. All in all this is very relaxing for the stressed feet.

WARTS

Because apple cider vinegar has an antibacterial effect and has a positive effect on the pH level of the skin, warts can also be successfully treated with apple cider vinegar. Apple cider vinegar inhibits the HPV virus through the malic acid it contains and also creates an alkaline environment. A property that contains the HPV virus. Ideally, mix 2 teaspoons of apple vinegar with a teaspoon of water and dab the solution on with a cotton pad. Simply place the damp cotton pad on the wart and fix it with a bandage or a plaster. After about two hours, remove the cotton pad and repeat the application daily. After some time, the wart will come off and fall off.

SUNBURN

Who does not long, especially after a long winter, for a bath in the sun. Of course, sunlight is very important for vitamin D production in the body. Unfortunately, the power of the sun is often underestimated and you burn faster than you thought. This does not mean that you should completely avoid the sun. Go into the sun and recharge your batteries, but make sure you have sufficient sun protection and avoid the midday sun. In case of sunburn, apple cider vinegar can be a good alternative to the classic Aloe Vera Gel. Depending on the affected skin areas, mix half a litre of cool water with half a cup of organic apple vinegar. Soak a cloth with the mixture and place it on the reddened skin areas. The water vinegar mixture cools the skin and the damaged skin layer is strengthened by the special ingredients. After a few minutes the application can be repeated as often as desired.

DEODORANT

As you already know, apple vinegar regulates the pH level of the skin and therefore also serves as a natural deodorant. Sometimes the smell of the vinegar can be disturbing and unpleasant, but it evaporates very quickly. Diluted with water it does not smell as strong anymore. For the application 2 tablespoons apple vinegar are diluted with 3 tablespoons water and applied with a cotton pad to the desired places (armpits, feet, etc.). The vinegar minimizes the sweat formation and binds the bacteria in the sweat.

ORAL CARE/BAD BREATH

The first priority of healthy oral hygiene is, of course, optimal dental care. Brushing your teeth twice a day, cleaning the interdental spaces with dental floss and cleaning your tongue is the basis of a healthy oral hygiene. In addition, a mouth shower and oil extraction can be a good idea. Chemical rinses, on the other hand, have a negative effect on the oral flora, allowing germs to spread much better. This in turn considerably increases the risk of bad breath. A mouthwash with apple cider vinegar, on the other hand, serves the oral flora and reduces the formation of sulphur. Rinse the mouth with a mixture of a tablespoon of naturally cloudy organic cider vinegar and a glass of water for 1 - 2 minutes. With regular use you will notice the positive difference. A nice side effect of the rinse is that discolourations on the teeth are reduced and thus whiter again.

SORE THROAT / HOARSENESS / COUGH

A cold, combined with sore throat, hoarseness and cough, is always unpleasant. Before you go to the pharmacy and buy overpriced medicines, fight the suffering with home remedies! In addition to many well-known household remedies, such as elderberry, ginger, salt solutions and lemon, etc., apple cider vinegar is particularly advisable due to its antimicrobial effect. The vinegar has a positive influence on the mucous membranes and helps therefore particularly well with a cold. To prevent the onset of a cold, it is advisable to add one to two tablespoons of organic apple vinegar daily to a glass of water and drink in the morning on an empty stomach. However, if the cold has already broken out, we recommend gargling with apple cider vinegar. Ideally you gargle every 2 hours with a mixture of 2 tablespoons apple vinegar, one tablespoon honey in a glass of warm water stirred. Due to the antibacterial and anti-inflammatory effect of honey and apple cider vinegar, the cold should quickly disappear into thin air.

HAEMORRHOIDS

You can reduce the unpleasant swelling of hemorrhoids with apple vinegar. Apple cider vinegar also has the ingenious property of decongesting and disinfecting and additionally promoting blood coagulation. To do this, carefully dab undiluted apple vinegar onto the itchy area with a small cotton pad. At first it will start to burn, but after a short time the itching is relieved and usually disappears completely. You will also notice that the swelling will decrease and the irritated area will heal.

SECTION 4: FURTHER CLEVER USES OF APPLE CIDER VINEGAR IN DAILY LIFE

In addition to the variety of applications for your health described above, apple cider vinegar is also a helpful companion in everyday life. Since it is so versatile, there are several other areas of application in the most diverse areas of everyday life. The following are just a few more examples.

APPLE CIDER VINEGAR AS A NATURAL CLEANING AGENT

Sometimes expensive household cleaners can be replaced with apple cider vinegar. So you save a lot of money and can also clean your home in an environmentally friendly way, because apple cider vinegar is free of harmful chemicals. Vinegar is an excellent cleaning agent for the household. Due to the acetic acid it is very well suited to remove stubborn grease, dirt and lime from the household. The vinegar also has a disinfectant effect and can therefore be used for cleaning kitchens, bathrooms and toilets. Apple cider vinegar is biodegradable and environmentally friendly. Nevertheless, it should not get into the eyes or hands of children.

To make a universal cleaning agent yourself, dilute apple vinegar 1:1 with water. You can also use pure vinegar to disinfect various surfaces.

Following some ideas where you can still use apple vinegar as a cleaning agent in the household.

Cleaning (disinfection) of refrigerator, oven, toilet etc.: Especially the application for the cleaning of the refrigerator is very suitable here, because apple vinegar works against mould and bad smells at the same time. Wipe your refrigerator (also seals!) regularly with vinegar water, bad smells and mould have no chance! Diluted apple vinegar can be used as an all-purpose cleaner in the whole household.

Descale the iron: Fill the iron with apple vinegar and steam. Then stand for several hours or leave to soak overnight if necessary. Finally rinse thoroughly.

Decalcify wash basins and water taps: Rub the calcified areas with apple vinegar water, leave on for 30 minutes and then rinse.

Descale the kettle: Fill the kettle with a little apple vinegar and let it boil. Leave to stand for 1-2 hours and rinse thoroughly.

Decalcify shower heads: Place in hot apple vinegar water for about 1 hour and leave to soak. The lime should then be completely dissolved.

Descaling the coffee machine: Fill the coffee machine with 1 glass of apple vinegar and let it run through. Then let it soak in for 2 hours and rinse thoroughly.

Lime stains on pots: First fill the pot with hot water, add 1 glass of apple cider vinegar and leave to soak for 2 hours. After the application all lime stains have disappeared.

Descale washing machine regularly: Pour a bottle of vinegar into the detergent chamber. Select the washing programme with the highest possible temperature and allow to take effect for approx. 30 minutes.

For me personally, the best application of vinegar is the cleaning of parquet or laminate floors. This allows you to effectively clean the wooden floor without leaving terrible marks on the surface. The reason for this is that vinegar has the perfect concentration of acetic acid (30%). Thus your floor becomes clean and there are no visible streaks on the surface. Cleaning products often contain chemical additives that can damage the floor. You can avoid this by using apple vinegar as a natural cleaning agent.

Before you start cleaning the wooden floor, make sure that all dust is removed. Dilute the vinegar with water in a ratio of 1 cup cider vinegar to 2 litres of water. Simply spread the vinegar water over the floor with a mop and wipe thoroughly. For stubborn stains you can also clean with undiluted vinegar. You don't have to worry about the smell, because it disappears after a short time. In addition, vinegar generally helps to neutralise unpleasant smells.

APPLE CIDER VINEGAR AS POLISHING AGENT

Another possible application of apple vinegar is its use as a polishing agent. If, for example, you want to clean silver, then mix half a cup of apple vinegar with 2 tablespoons of baking powder and place the silver to be polished in the cleaning solution for about half an hour. After the contact time, simply rinse the silver with water. Other metals such as brass, copper or stainless steel can be cleaned and polished with a paste of salt and vinegar in a ratio of 1:1. Apply the cleaning paste to the above-mentioned metal objects and let it take effect. After about an hour, rinse with water and allow to dry.

LAUNDRY

Spray dirty laundry with apple cider vinegar before washing and let it react for one night. This makes it easier to remove the dirt when washing. Sweat marks on T-shirts or shirts can be removed very easily by soaking them overnight with apple vinegar and then washing them afterwards. A reason for sometimes rough or hard laundry is limy water. If you now add pure, undiluted apple vinegar to the chamber for the fabric softener, your laundry will become soft and pleasantly cuddly again.

Do you know it? White laundry gets a grayish veil over time. This can have several causes. Incorrect dosage of the detergent can cause detergent residue to be responsible for the grey haze. If you use too little detergent, dirt particles can remain in the fibres and form a grey haze. Another reason may be that water containing lime is responsible for the grey haze. Solution: Soak your laundry in vinegar water! Either in a bucket overnight or via the pre-wash function of your washing machine. Simply add vinegar to the appropriate compartment of the washing machine instead of detergent.

To freshen up laundry and remove unpleasant odours, you can also put vinegar water (equal parts of vinegar and water) in a spray bottle and spray the garment with it. At first it will smell unpleasant, but this smell disappears very quickly and then all bad smells will have disappeared. Besides, creases and wrinkles will have disappeared.

CLEANING THE CARPET

Professional carpet cleaning is expensive and very time-consuming. You can also simply clean your short pile carpet yourself and refresh the colours with vinegar water. Mix in a bucket, water and vinegar in a ratio of approx. 1:10, i.e. approx. one bottle of apple vinegar on one bucket of water.

Before you start to clean the carpet, it should be well vacuumed. Ideally, use a lint-free cotton cloth for the scrubber. Rub the carpet with the moistened cloth. Do not exert too much pressure on the scrubbing brush. Too much pressure would push the dirt too much into the carpet fabric and would not be washed out completely. After the treatment you will see how fresh the colours shine again!

OTHER ADDITIONAL APPLICATIONS

- Washing fruit and vegetables: To wash fruit and vegetables you simply dip apples etc. into a mixture of 1:1 water and apple vinegar to destroy bacteria and other germs.

- Ant control: Because ants have a very good sense of smell and do not like strong odours, apple vinegar helps especially well. Simply drizzle some vinegar into the areas where the ants occur. From now on the ants will avoid the areas covered with vinegar.

- Mosquitoes and ticks: Apple cider vinegar mixed with some water can help fight mosquitoes both indoors and outdoors with this simple remedy. Place the mixture in a bowl as close as possible to where you are. Apple vinegar is also an excellent household remedy against ticks. Mix the apple cider vinegar in equal parts with water and then apply to the affected area with a cloth or cotton ball. The vinegar relieves pain, redness and disinfects the surrounding skin.

- Flowers: Cut flowers stay fresh much longer if you add two tablespoons apple cider vinegar and two tablespoons sugar to the flower vase.

- Insect bites: Apple cider vinegar has a decongestant and cooling effect, relieves itching and helps to dissolve insect venom. Apply apple cider vinegar to the painful area as soon as possible after the sting and repeat as necessary.

- Against unpleasant room odours: Basically vinegar has a disinfecting effect and helps against unpleasant odours. Simply mix vinegar with water in a mixing ratio of 1:1. When the vinegar odor has disappeared, it has neutralized the other odors as well. In most cases one application is sufficient, only in case of very strong odours you should repeat the process after some time.

- Wallpaper stripper: To remove old wallpaper from the walls, you do not need a special wallpaper stripper from the DIY store. It is enough to mix apple vinegar with water and apply this mixture generously to the old wallpaper with a large brush. This makes it easy to remove them from the wall.

- Windows streak-free: Simply add a good dash of apple vinegar to the cleaning water for the windows and they will be streak-free clean. The vinegar helps to loosen the dirt and prevents limescale deposits from the cleaning water from accumulating on the window pane.

- Mould: A very good application against mould is,

how could it be otherwise, apple vinegar! The acetic acid kills the mold, whereby it dissolves, and you can remove it afterwards effortlessly. If you have spots of mould, wipe them carefully with apple cider vinegar or let them work into apple cider vinegar. Then it is very easy to remove the mould from the surfaces.

SECTION 5: MAKE YOUR OWN APPLE CIDER VINEGAR YOURSELF

Apple cider vinegar from the supermarket is very cheap. But if you want a pure organic product, you can simply make your own cider vinegar. The homemade apple cider vinegar is of course the healthiest form of apple cider vinegar you can consume. Often you will find organic apple cider vinegar only in special organic shops and are often not to be found in other shops at all. Fortunately, it is very easy to make your own cider vinegar, just be patient. In the following I would like to describe the different possibilities to you to production.

APPLE CIDER VINEGAR FROM THE APPLE SHELL AND KERNEL HOUSING

Ingredients:

- Apple shells and cores

- Water

Leave the apple leftovers in the air until they are browned by the oxygen. Then rinse a glass container with hot water to prevent the growth of bacteria.

Now pour the apple remains into a glass with a wide opening and fill it with boiled and cooled water until all apple pieces are completely covered. Finally, simply cover the glass with a cloth and let it rest in a dark and warm place. Make sure that the glass is not exposed to sunlight. No lid is used as the fermentation process requires air to breathe.

The contents will thicken after about three days and a

brownish foam will appear on the surface. This is an indication of the beginning of the fermentation process.

Stir the mixture every day with a clean spoon to prevent mould from forming on the surface. After about 1 to 2 weeks you will notice the typical vinegar smell. After the waiting time, the vinegar mother develops on the surface. This can also be used for the next fermentation process to speed up the process. Let the glass rest for about a month until you test the vinegar. If the taste is not strong enough for you, you can leave it to stand for a while. Finally, simply pour the vinegar through a cloth or sieve and pour into a tightly sealable, ideally dark, bottle. The cider vinegar is now ready and can be used.

PRODUCTION OF APPLE CIDER VINEGAR FROM APPLE JUICE

Ingredients:

- 5 litres of apple juice (ideally freshly pressed from organic apples)

- 1 bottle of pure yeast

- 1 yeast nutrient salt tablet

- 500 ml vinegar mother

- Fermenter with fermenting attachment

- bulbous glass jar

First of all, the fresh apple juice must be fermented. This is where the cider is produced.

The difference between the vinegar fermentation described above and the wine fermentation is the oxygen.

With wine fermentation this takes place without oxygen supply. A fermentation balloon with a bent and water-filled fermentation tube is therefore absolutely necessary. To produce the wine from the apple juice, the apple juice is filled into the fermentation balloon and the pure yeast is added. Dissolve the yeast nutrition salt tablet in a glass with a little water and then add it to the fermentation container. Fill the balloon to about two thirds so that there is still enough space for the gases produced during fermentation. Immediately after filling, the container must be closed with the fermenting attachment and placed in a dry place at a constant temperature (not above 22°C).

The fermentation process takes about 4 weeks. You can see this by the fact that no more bubbles will rise in the fermentation tube. The resulting cider must be poured through a coffee filter to produce a clear wine from the cloudy cider. The vinegar mother is needed so that the vinegar can now be produced from the cider. Generally applies: per 1 litre of wine about 100ml vinegar mother.

You already know how the vinegar mother is made. You can use it wonderfully for the process of making apple vinegar. Pour the cider into a bulbous glass container and add the vinegar mother. To allow the oxygen necessary for the vinegar fermentation to penetrate, close the container with a cotton ball only. Finally, place the glass in a warm place so that the vinegar bacteria can take effect. Now it takes about one to two weeks until the cider vinegar is ready for bottling. You will recognize this by the fact that the vinegar has a sour smell. Now you should let the apple cider vinegar ripen for another two months in a cool place. After this time you can enjoy it. As already said, please bring patience with you. However, it is worth it in any case, because your self-produced apple cider vinegar cannot be replaced with any vinegar from the supermarket.

I would like to show you that there are a lot of variations to make apple vinegar yourself. Therefore here is another possibility.

APPLE CIDER VINEGAR FROM BRANDY VINEGAR

Ingredients:

- 1 litre brandy vinegar

- 4 apples

Peel and core the apples. Then cut into small pieces and place in a bulbous container. Fill the jar with brandy vinegar and close it. Let it steep for 2 to 3 weeks in a cool place and already after 3 weeks you can enjoy the apple vinegar. The apple remains on the bottom let the vinegar ripen further and are a great indication of which vinegar it is.

SECTION 6: RECIPES WITH APPLE CIDER VINEGAR

MAGIC DRINK FOR YOUR HEALTH

- consists of: water, apple vinegar, lemon and cranberry juice

Effect:

- Supports the digestion

- Regulates the blood sugar level

- Has an antioxidant effect

- Filter system for liver and kidneys

- Regulates the cholesterol level

- Harmonisation of blood lipid levels

- anti-inflammatory effect

It is best to use lukewarm water, as this water comes closest to our body temperature and therefore has a very supportive effect on digestion.

Continue by taking half a lemon and squeezing it out. Take high quality apple vinegar and cranberry juice. The cranberry juice should ideally be the mother juice, naturally cloudy and without added sugar.

- 100-200ml warm water

- juice of half a lemon

- 1-2 teaspoons apple cider vinegar

- 1-2 teaspoons cranberry juice

Mix everything well together and consume the drink every morning on an empty stomach. Of course it can be consumed throughout the day. Ideally before meals.

Try to make it a habit to drink every day.

HEALTHY APPLE VINEGAR HONEY DRINK

The fastest all-round drink for every morning is the "Good Morning Power Drink"!

Simply mix 1 glass of water with 2 teaspoons of apple vinegar and 1-2 teaspoons of honey.

Drink this power drink every morning on an empty stomach in small sips to start the day healthy and fit.

CONCLUSION: APPLE VINEGAR IS A JACK-OF-ALL-TRADES!

Apple cider vinegar is a cheap and above all valuable household remedy which you can use daily.

Whether for your health, as cosmetic or medical product and even as cleaning agent in the household - hardly any other substance can be used as versatile as apple cider vinegar. And the most beautiful thing about it: This natural jack-of-all-trades helps for a healthy well-being!

Thank you very much for your time!

Printed in Poland
by Amazon Fulfillment
Poland Sp. z o.o., Wrocław